Care of the Hip Spica Cast

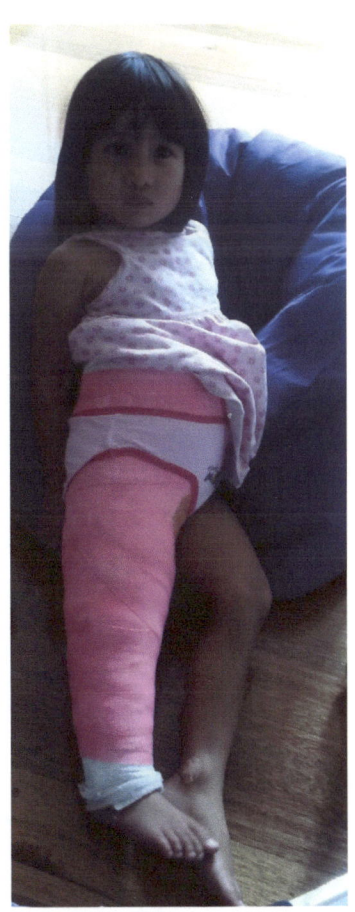

Written By
Robyn Lambert

DEDICATION

To my beautiful man and gorgeous children, thank you for all your love and support.

ACKNOWLEDGEMENT

Image on page 28 is of a GoGirl TM toileting aid. For interest in the GoGirl products go to
https://go-girl.com/how-to-get-gogirl/

TABLE OF CONTENTS

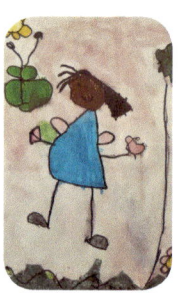

INTRODUCTION

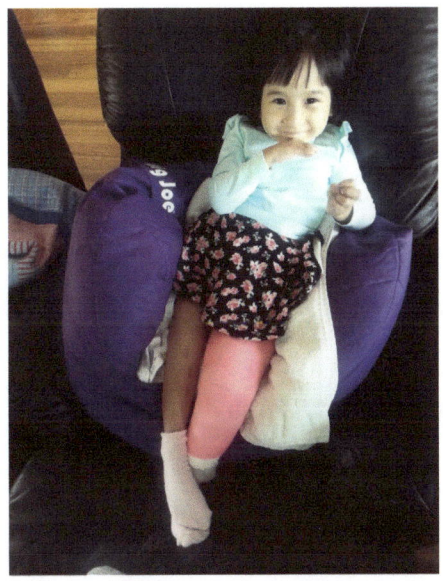

TIP! BEFORE BEGINNING ANY TASKS,
TAKE A DEEP BREATH IN AND SLOWLY LET IT OUT.

LET ALL YOUR STRESS GO BECAUSE THAT IS THE LAST
THING YOU NEED RIGHT NOW. DO THIS OFTEN AND YOU
WILL BE FINE.

ALL TECHNIQUES IN THIS BOOK CAN BE USED FOR BOTH BOYS AND GIRLS

When surgery is performed on the hip or thigh area, sometimes it necessitates the wearing of a hip spica cast to keep the child from moving while these areas heal. Immediately after surgery the cast can be tight due to swelling. Indeed some casts need to be cut around the upper abdomen or leg areas to accommodate this swelling. This is usually done by the doctor or nursing staff in hospital. The swelling eventually subsides and the cast becomes looser, particularly if the child loses weight post-surgery. This book is about care of the hip spica at home, keeping it as clean as possible and reducing odour that is usually associated with casts being on for a long time. It also provides many tips on keeping your child comfortable. The main focus is on babies, toddlers and pre-school children, however, the ideas in this book may be adapted to suit older children.

TIP! The advice in this book may also be adapted for use in Day Care, Pre-school or Kindergarten settings.

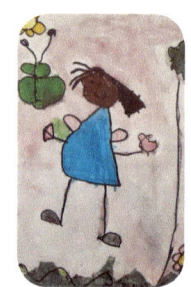

LIFTING YOUR CHILD

You will have to learn to become very good at lifting your child with the hip spica cast on. You will need to move them from the bed to the stroller or wheelchair; or to the toilet or washing area. In all cases below it should be said that lifting a child of any size with a hip spica on, can put you at risk of a back injury. Hip spica casts are very heavy and can add many kilograms to your child's weight.

SAFETY TIP! If you suffer from a bad back it might be beneficial to seek professional advice on lifting prior to your child's surgery. Your therapist may have ideas that will suit your individual needs.

SAFETY TIP! Correct lifting techniques will help prevent injury from happening.

SAFETY TIP! Due to the weight of the hip spica, never lift your child up by the arms or shoulders as it could result in injury to those areas.

BABIES, TODDLERS AND PRE-SCHOOLERS

First and foremost you must enlist the help of the child wherever possible. This solves two problems-

- To help you lift them successfully, preventing injury to either yourself or your child and
- To teach them how to move about in a bed or chair and to make themselves comfortable

Of course this is not going to happen with a baby. You are the only one that knows your child's level of understanding so give it a go with a toddler. They may astound you with what they can achieve with a little prompting.

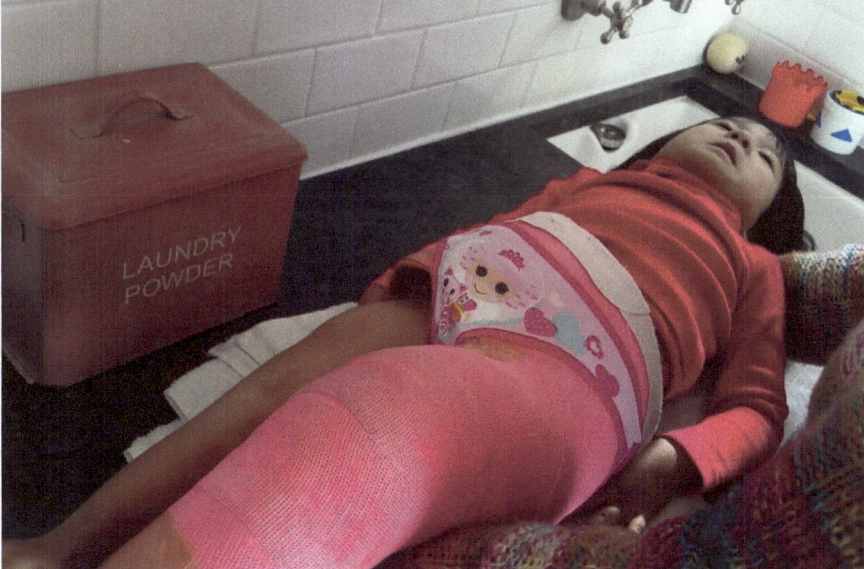

SAFETY TIP! Bend your knees, lean forward by bending at the hips but keep your back straight. Slide your arms, up to the inside of your elbow area, both under the child's knees and under the shoulder blade area furthest from you.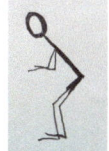

SAFETY TIP! Do NOT hunch over.

3

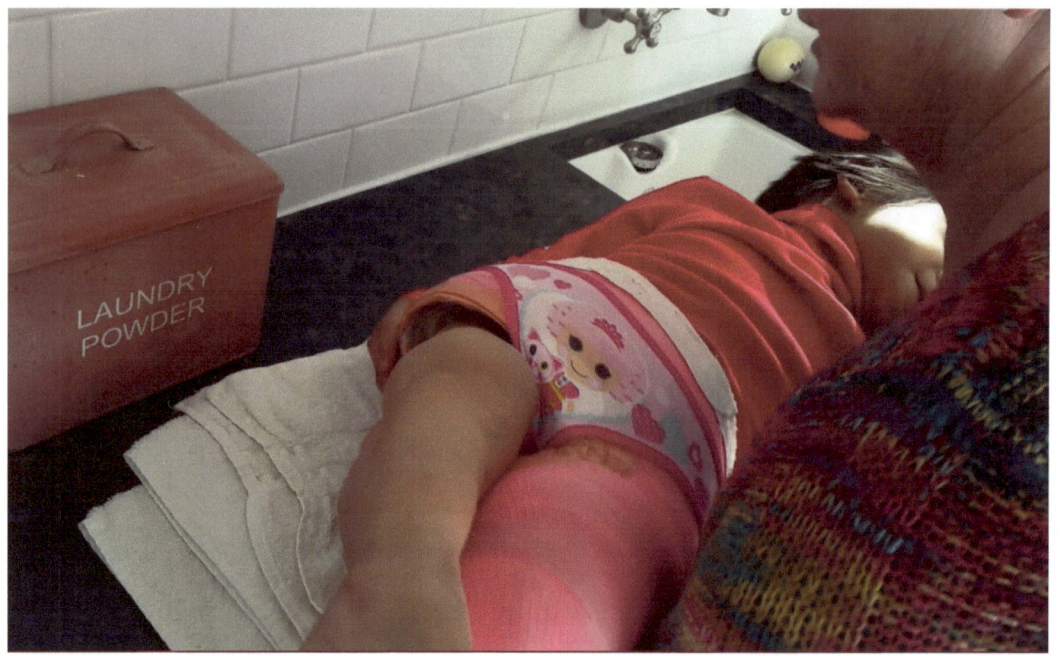

Instead of pulling or dragging the child to you, draw your hands and forearms toward your body and the child will roll toward your chest area. If your child is old enough to understand and can help, get them to roll towards you.

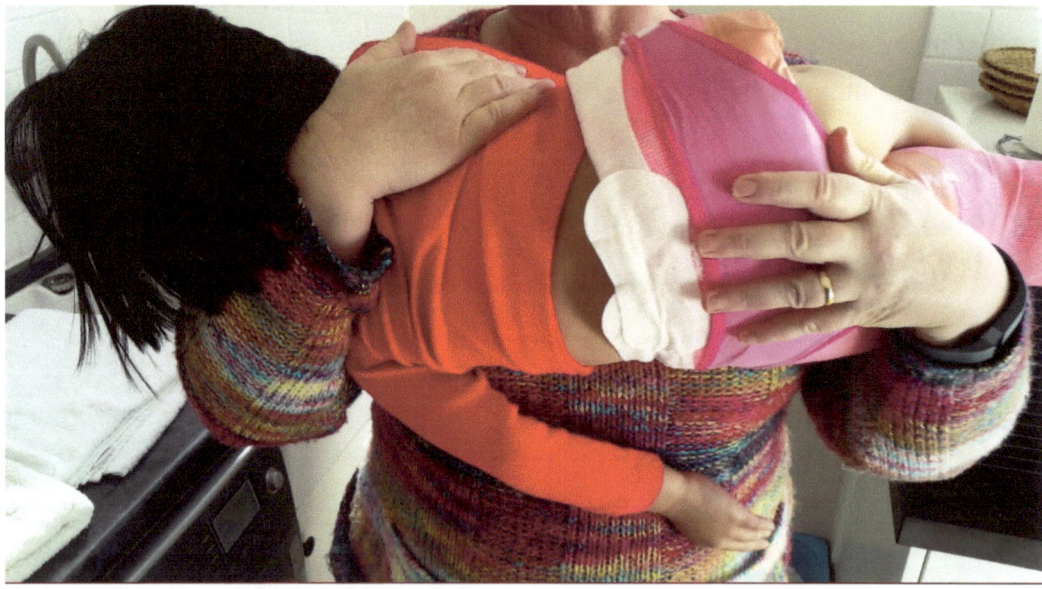

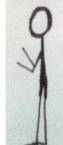 Straighten your legs to stand up bringing your forward leaning straight back into the vertical position. Hold your child close to your chest. The front of their body should be in contact with your chest. Remember push up and straighten your legs rather than lifting with your arms.

When putting your child down,lower yourself by bending your knees, still keeping your back straight, unroll your arms and let them slowly roll back on to the area.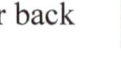

SAFETY TIP! Ensure you don't hunch over or lean forward when carrying your child. Maintain a straight posture whilst walking to the area you are taking your child to.

SAFETY TIP! Before moving, clear the path of where you are taking your child. The last thing you want is to trip over a toy or shoe whilst carrying your child.

BIGGER CHILDREN

It is important that you teach your child very quickly how to move about with a hip spica on. They will need to know how to move from the bed to the wheelchair and then to the toilet/washing space, with little to no help.

It is essential that your child maintain a sense of control over their situation as a way of not feeling helpless. They need to feel that they can do what they did before but adapted to their current situation; for example –

- Wheeling themselves in their wheelchair
- Transferring themselves to the toilet and back to the wheelchair when finished
- Washing, dressing and grooming themselves with little or no intervention.
  Making themselves comfortable in bed or on a chair

Children are enormously resilient and often do better than adults in these situations. They only need to be shown how and will often want to do it on their own from then on. Children love a challenge and to feel grown up. Being cared for like a baby can be demoralizing for them and counterproductive to their healing process. Self-care makes for a happier child, so independence is the key.

If your child hasn't already been shown how to do these tasks by the hospital, then you must seek help from either a physiotherapist or occupational therapist to show the best way to do them. It might be an idea to contact the hospital where your child will be having their surgery and find out if this is going to be taught before going home. If not, then look for a therapist who will show you and your child the relevant techniques and attend a session together. At first your child might find these tasks difficult but in a very short time they will develop amazing upper body strength.

If these steps are not taken and you constantly lift your bigger/older child, then you are at huge risk of injuring your back and will not be able to help your child at all. Teaching them to help themselves will make everyone happy.

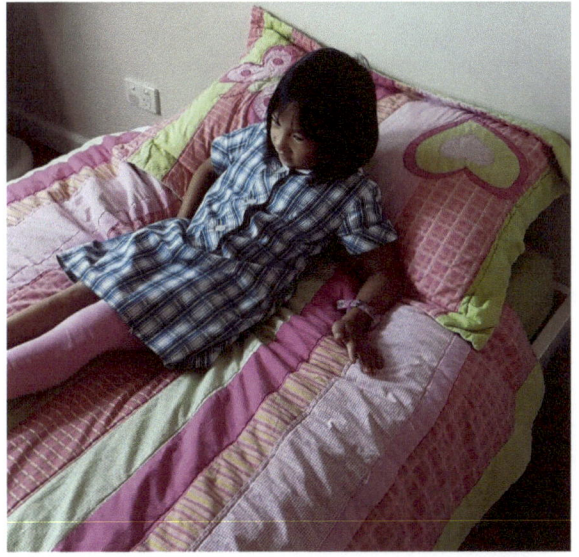

Moving about the bed independently

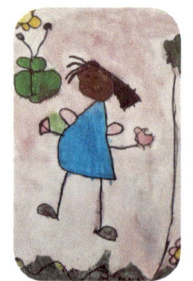

WASHING YOUR CHILD

If you are going to wash or to toilet your child, make sure you take all the equipment and supplies that you need for the task before you bring your child to those areas.

ITEMS NEEDED PRIOR TO BRINGING YOUR CHILD TO THE WASH AREA

- You will need two towels folded (old ones are ok)

- Another towel for warmth and to dry with

- Wash cloths 2 - 3 (or more if you prefer)

- Moisturiser

- Small rubbish bag

- Packet of Panty liners

- Packet of incontinence pads

- Nappy (if required)

- Shampoo and body wash (baby wash is perfect for all ages and can be used for hair and body)

- Plastic cup

- Child's clothing

- Perhaps a small toy or book to distract your child if they become restless

SAFETYTIP! Once you bring your child to the wash area you cannot leave them unattended.

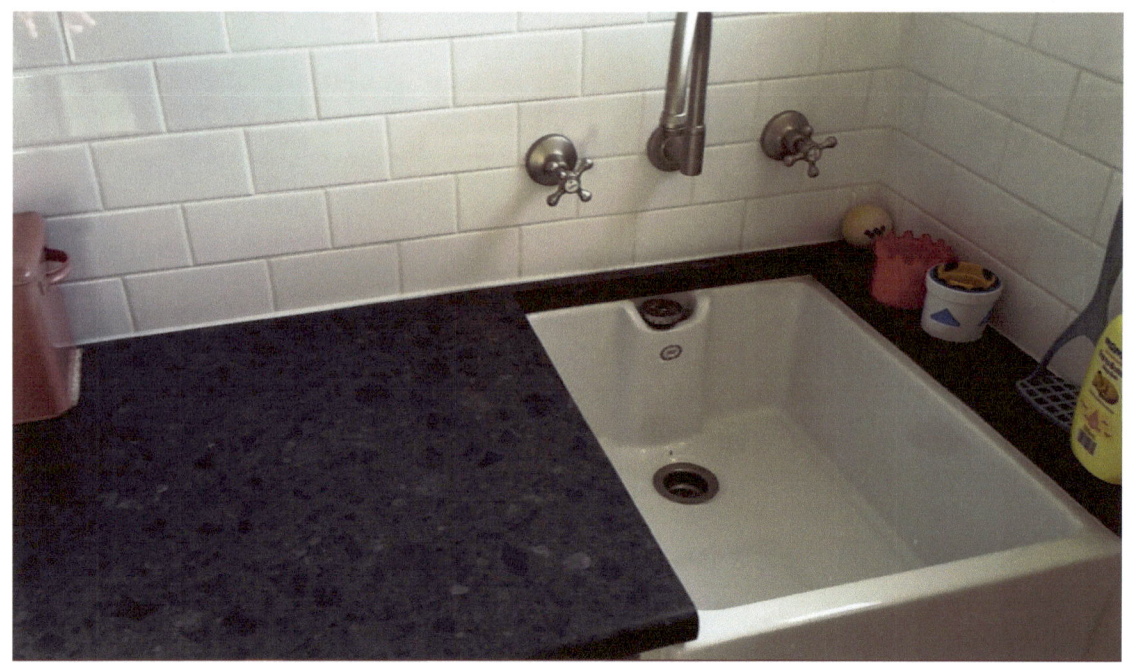

Any area that is of a comfortable height to work at such as a kitchen bench, laundry bench (pictured), even a washing machine top will work, as long as these surfaces are directly beside a sink. Have a cup handy by the sink so you can use it to wet and rinse your child's hair.

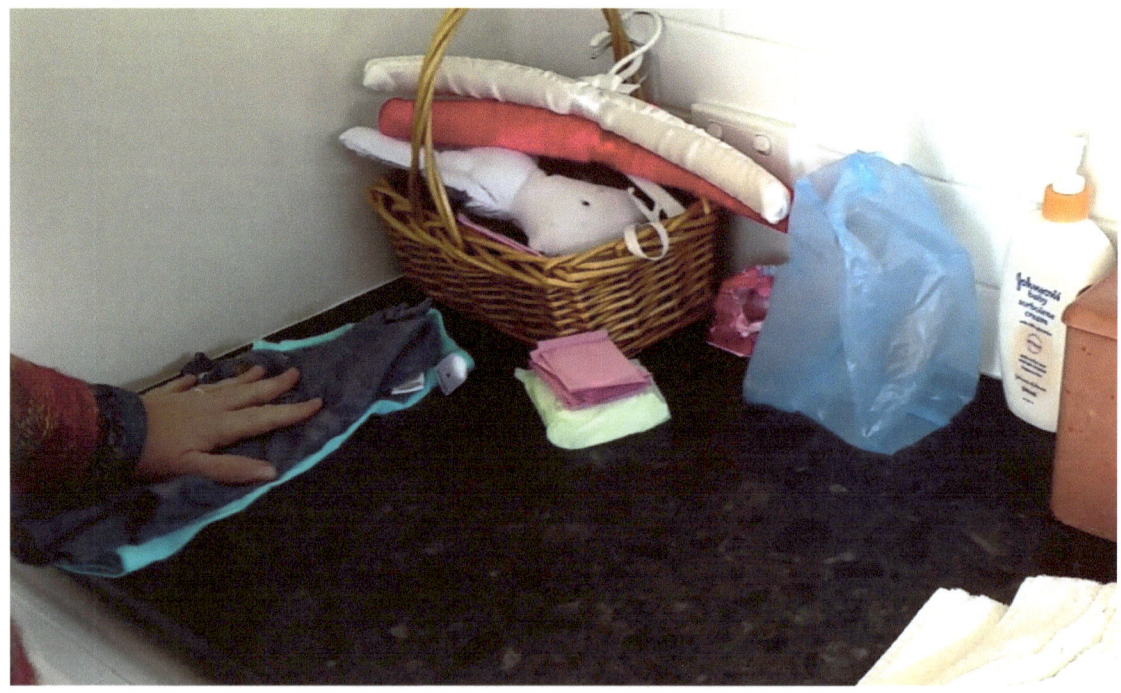

Ensure you have all the materials and equipment you will need prior to bringing your child to be washed as you won't be able to go and get it once you have begun the wash. Have a rubbish bag handy to put all soiled nappies or old pads and wrappers in. Have moisturizer ready for any dry spots that you notice.

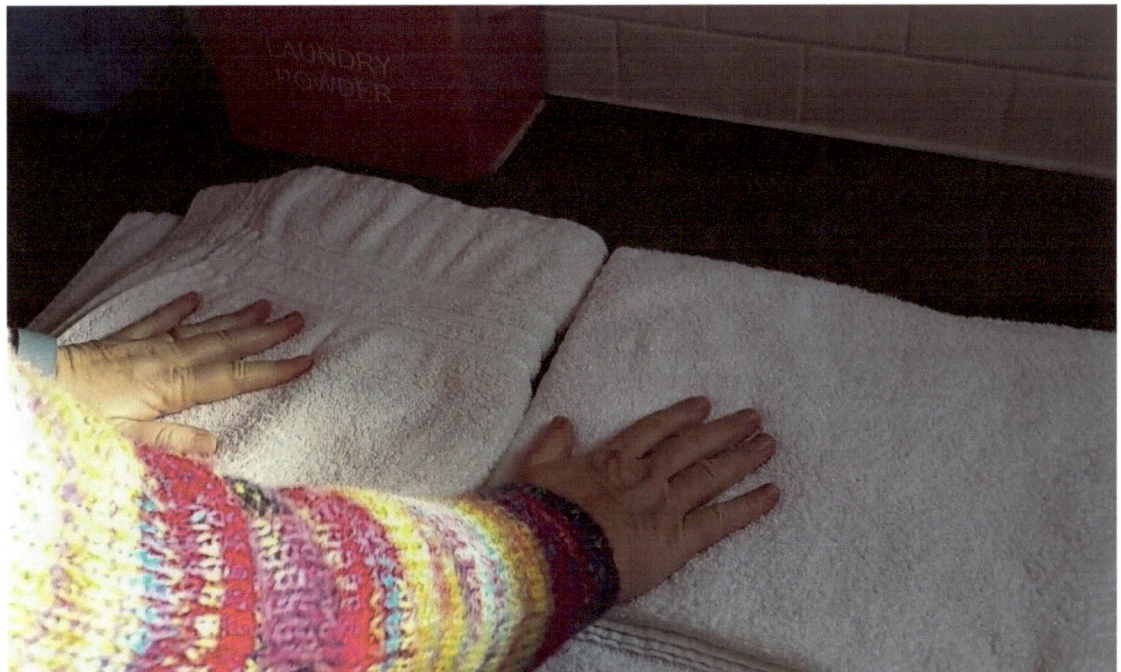

Put two towels down to lay your child on during the wash. This acts as both a soft padded surface to lie on and to absorb water from underneath your child.

SAFETY TIP! A padded nappy change mat, with raised sides, can be placed under the towels for extra comfort. However, do not rely on it to prevent your baby from falling.

SAFETY TIP! Always keep at least one hand on your child when they are in the washing area

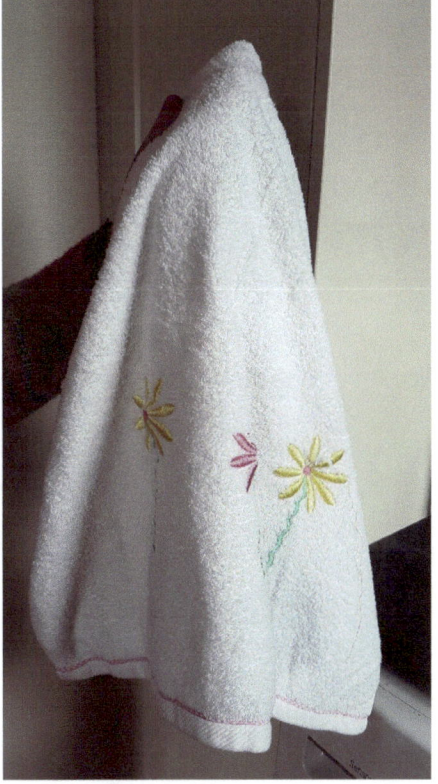

Have a third towel to cover your child so they won't get cold. You can then use this towel to dry them when they are washed.

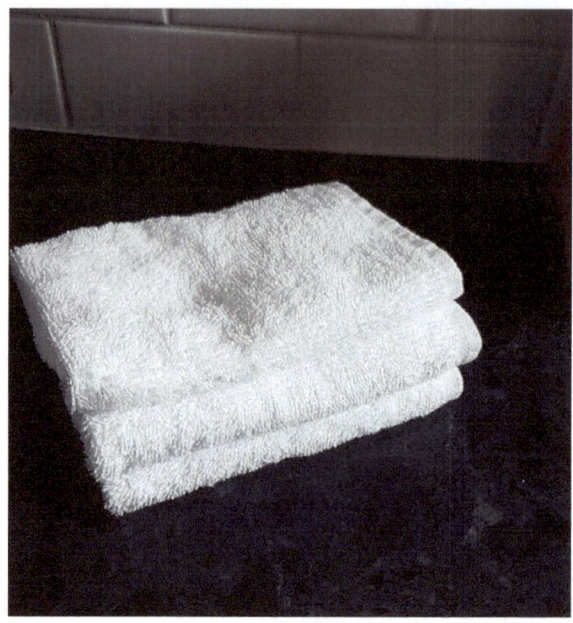

TIP! Have a number of wash cloths handy so you can have a clean one each for the face and body, groin and bottom areas.

Once you are ready you can go and get your child and bring them to the wash area. Undress your child, remove their nappy, if they have one, and dispose in the rubbish bag. Cover your child with a towel to keep warm.

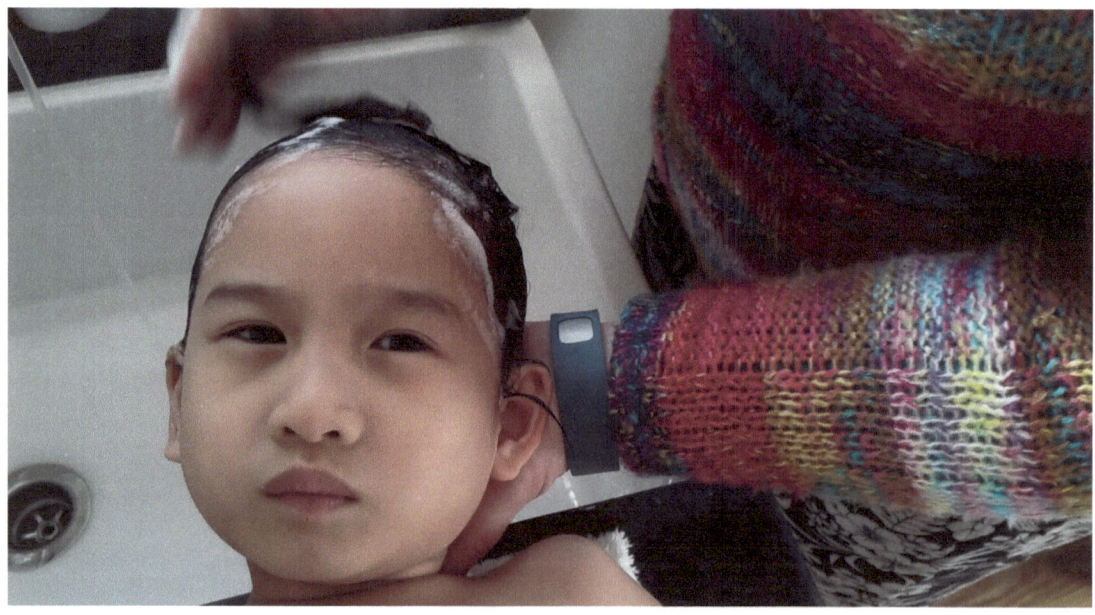

With one hand resting on the child to stabilize, start to run your water to the desired temperature.

SAFETY TIP! Leave the water running but make sure the tap is out of the way of your child.

Use the towels they are lying on to slide your child's head over the sink or basin. Tuck the excess towel under the neck but maintain support of their head throughout the washing of the hair. Alternately you can lift them along using the lifting technique described earlier, and not tuck the towel under.

SAFETY TIP! Support your child's head the whole time you are washing the hair. Use one hand under the head and wash with the other.

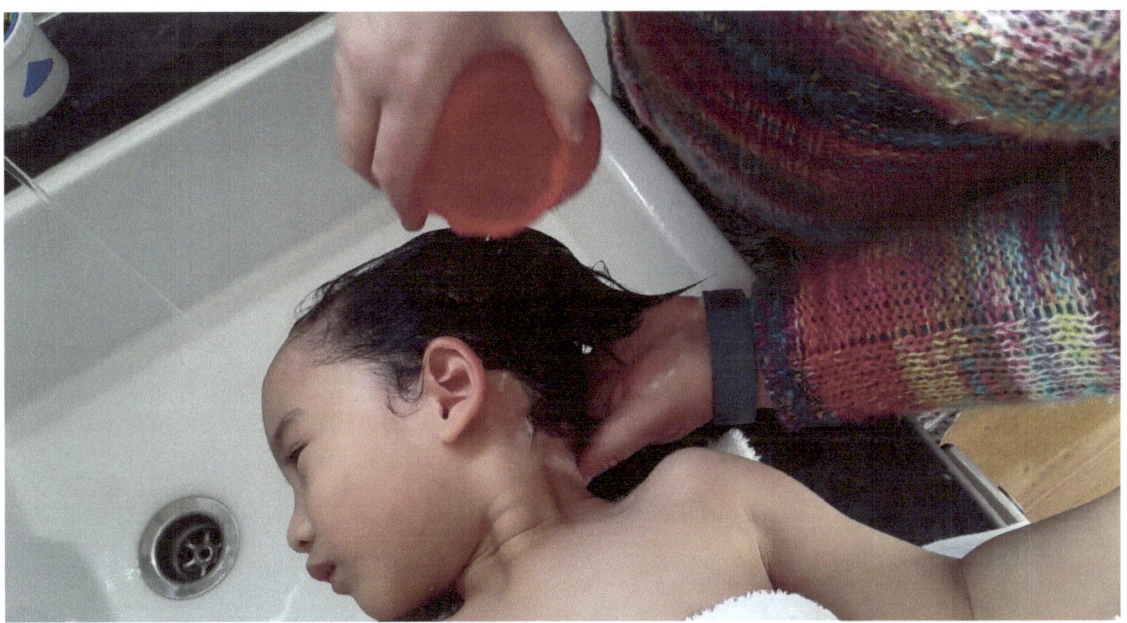

With their head slightly tilted backward pour water using the cup over your child's hair. If your child is able to understand and help, get them to turn their head from side to side making it easier for you to wash their hair.

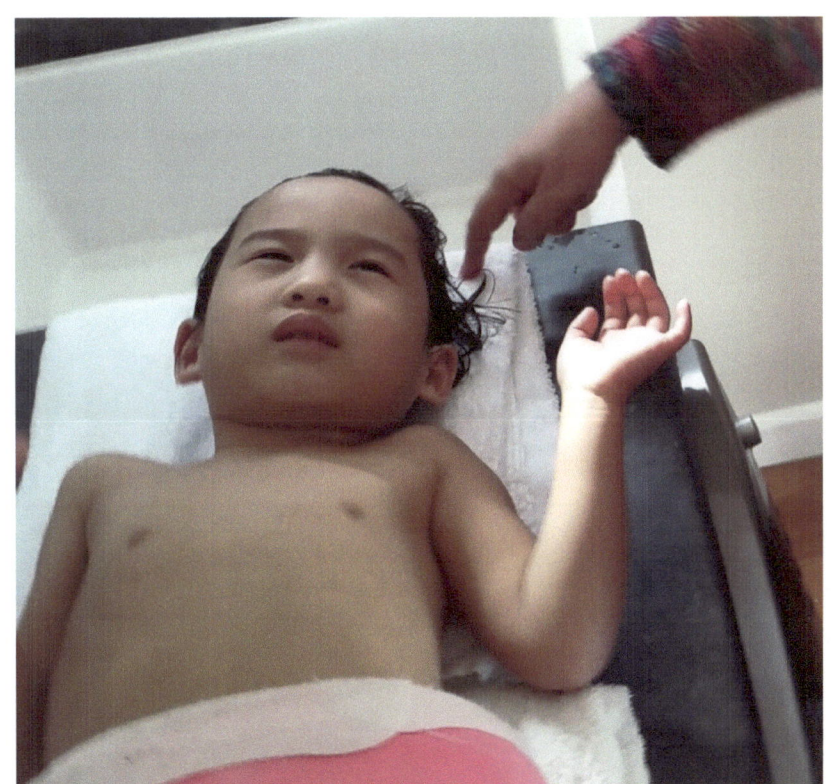

Slide your child back onto the bench, unfolding the excess towel that was under their neck as you go or lift them back using the lifting technique. There is no need to dry their hair at this point with the towel as water from their head will absorb into the folded towel underneath them.

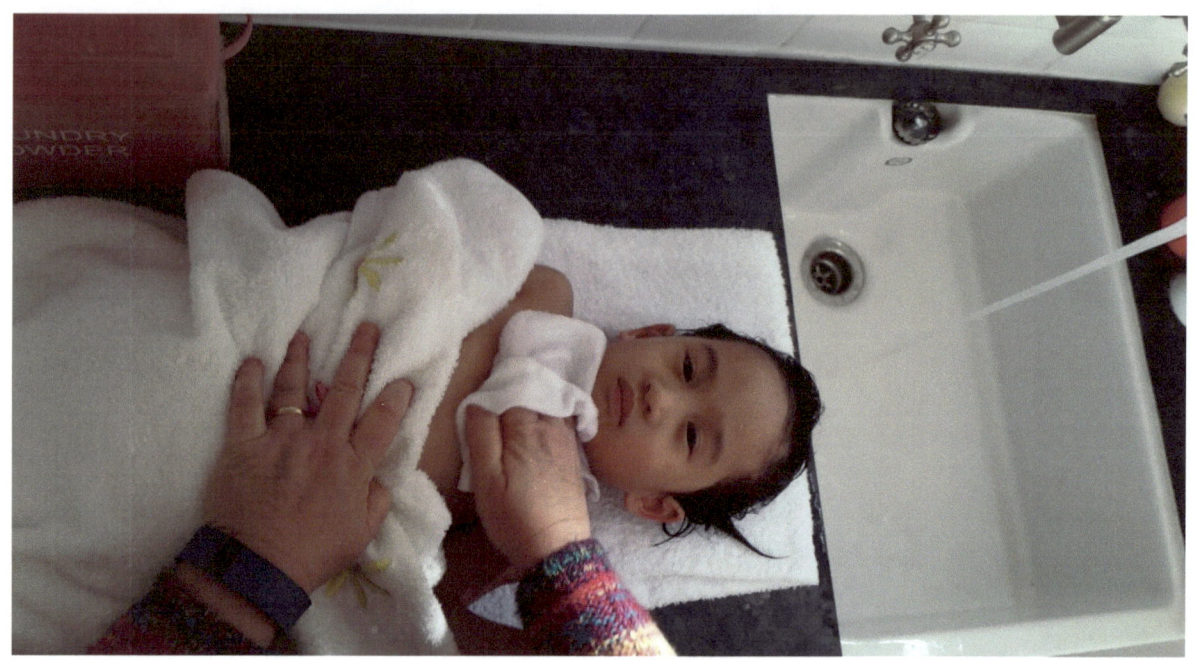

Wash the body by only exposing small areas at a time. For example, start with the face, creases round the neck, the chest, arms and armpits.

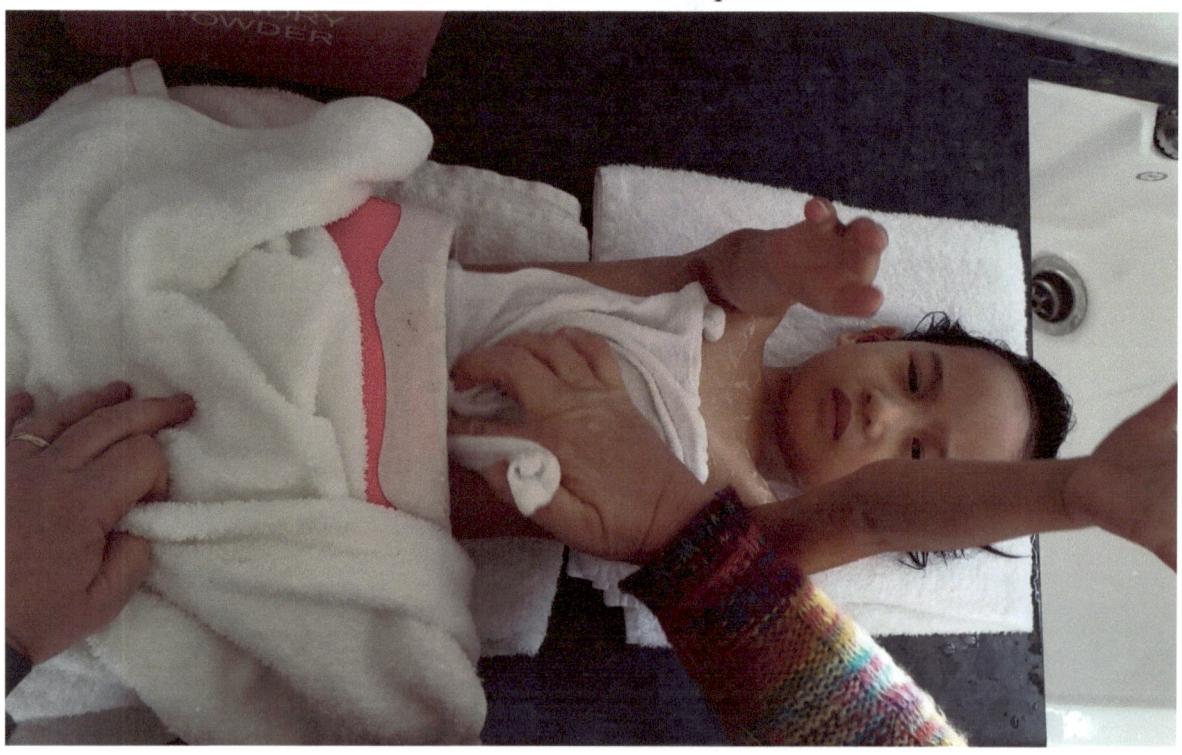

Wash slightly under the cast if you have room to do this but go no further than the second joint of your fingers (pictured). Dry thoroughly. DO NOT force your hand under the cast at any point if it is too tight.

SAFETY TIP! It may be tempting to clean the wound site if you can see it as there may be a dressing soaked in blood or old blood near the wound but it is paramount to AVOID THE WOUND as you risk it opening up. If a dressing has come free on its own, only then can you remove it. No dressing needs to replace it so DO NOT attempt it.

SAFETY TIP! If you can see that the wound and it has opened, contact your doctor or surgeon immediately.

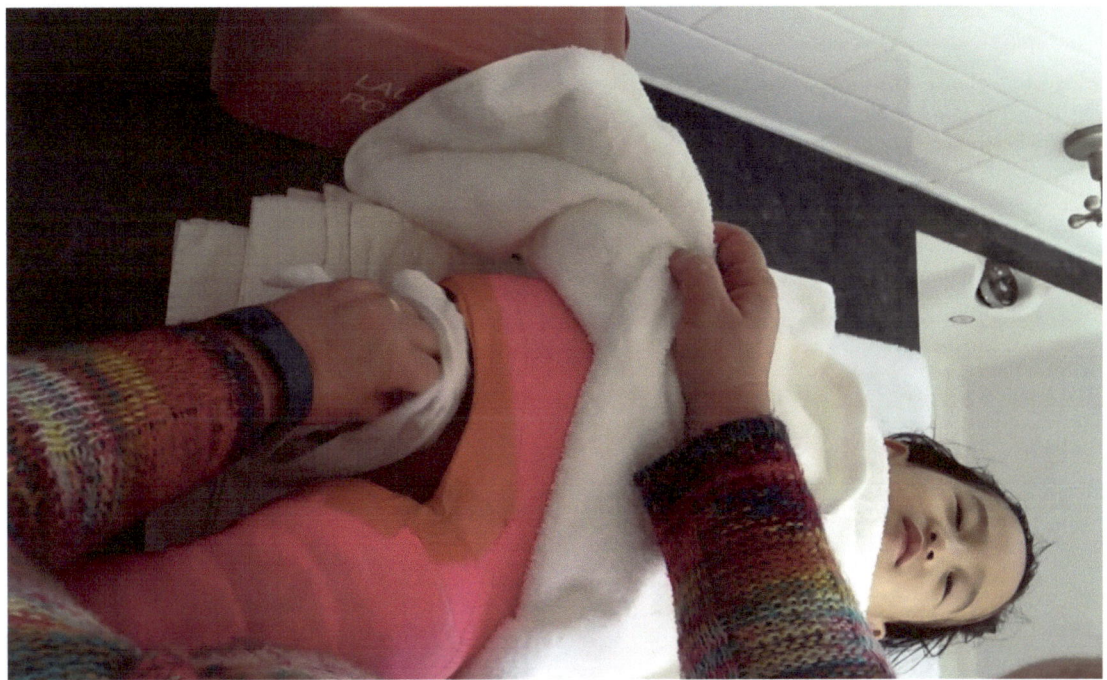

Do the same when washing around the groin area. Only wash a small way in. Dry thoroughly. Continue with washing the legs and that are not covered by the cast. Dry thoroughly.

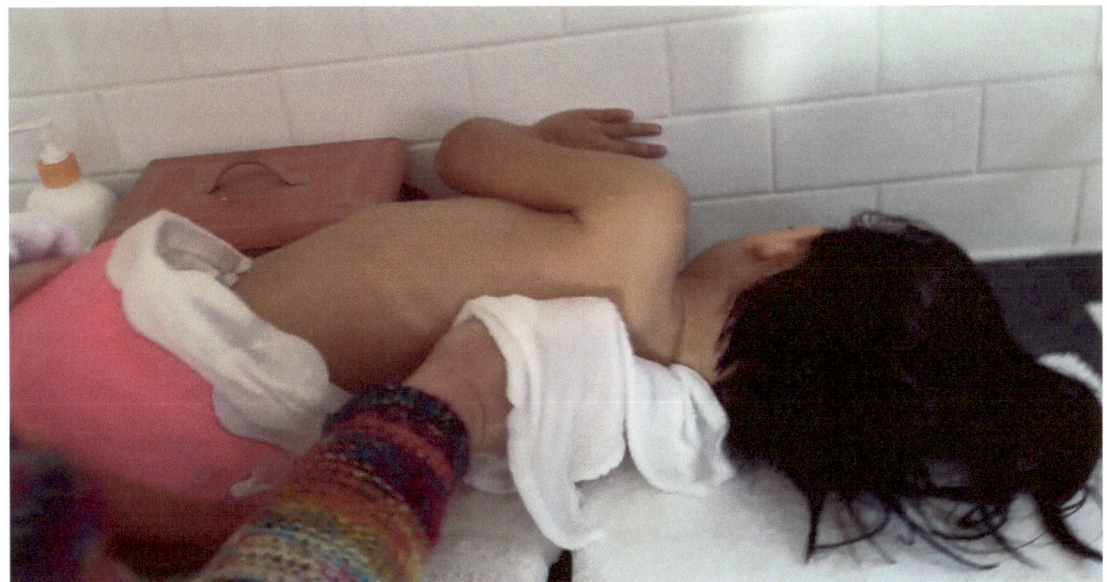

Encourage your child to roll to the wall so you can wash their back. As your child spends quite a bit of time on their back, they sweat more in this area. Make sure you clean thoroughly as this can cause itching and discomfort. There is no need to dry their back as rolling back on to the folded towels will do this job for you. Now wash their bottom area thoroughly, being careful not to put your hand too far under the cast.

SAFETY TIP! Ensure each area is thoroughly dried before moving on to the next area. As the children are not moving around much, air flow around creased areas on their body is reduced. If areas such as armpits and neck creases for example, stay damp after a wash, it may lead to skin breakdown.

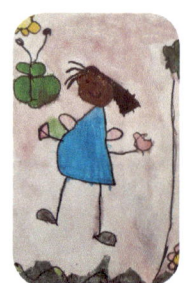

APPLYING WATERPROOF TAPE

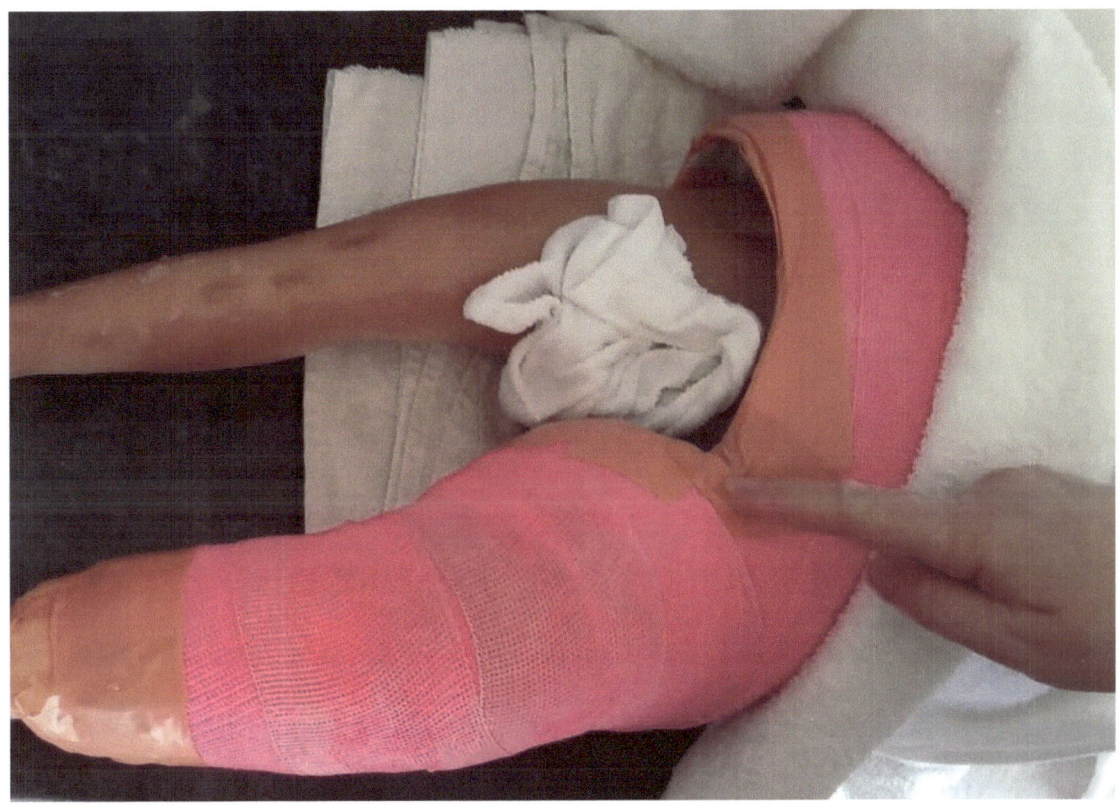

As soon as you are able, either in the hospital or as soon as you get home, apply a waterproof medical tape such as the tape in the picture. Apply to the raw edges of the groin, bottom and ankle area or where ever your cast extends down to.

The tape is applied to the pictured areas as the raw plaster is exposed. Even though the outside of the plaster may be covered in fiberglass (as pictured here), the edges are still plaster and as such tend to be sharp. The plaster can crumble and become soft if it gets wet with water or urine. The crumbling plaster also comes off in bed and is very itchy when in contact with skin. Always replace the tape as soon as it starts to peel off as it may wrinkle up and cause irritation and discomfort.

TIP! Some hospitals will offer you a roll of the waterproof tape to take home. If they don't offer, ask. You may not get a "yes" but it doesn't hurt to ask. It is freely available to purchase at pharmacies. It can be expensive but it is worth it.

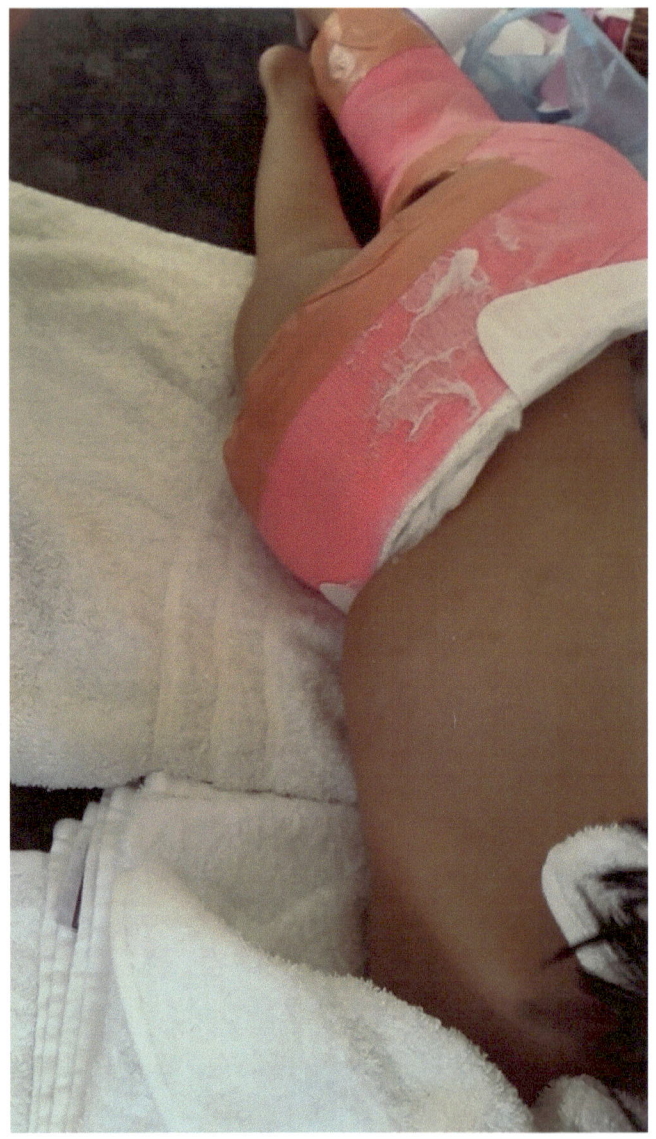

Taping around the buttock area is to protect the cast from urine and faeces as well as the sharp edge. Remember to remove any tape that starts to peel and replace it.

You can tape the top of the cast near the abdomen/chest area if you wish; however, the tape can be expensive to buy. It is probably a less expensive option to use the panty liner method, used in the next section, for lining the top of the cast. Keep the tape for areas that are more prone to soiling, wetness and crumbling such as groin, buttocks and ankles.

PROTECTING SKIN FROM CAST EDGES

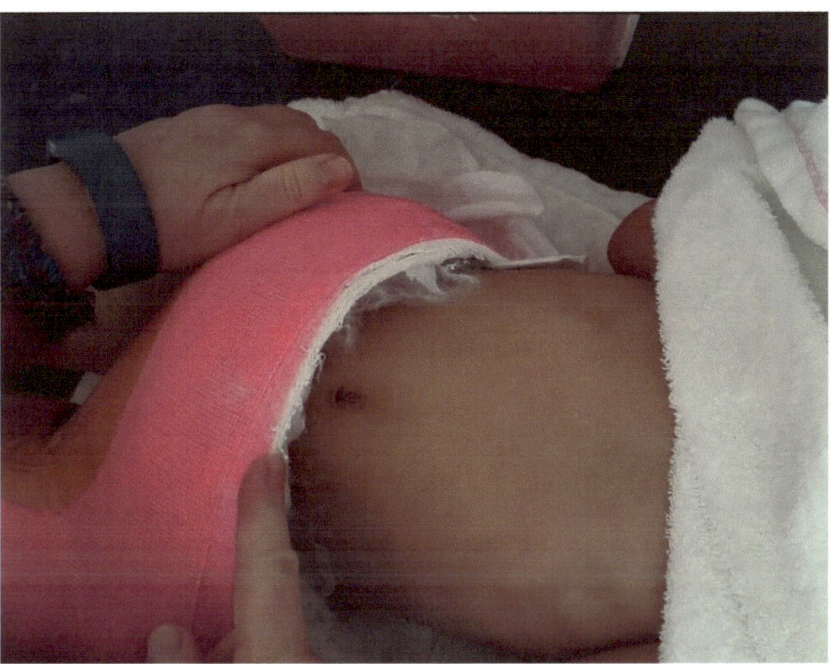

The top of the cast can be very sharp and jagged. When your child sits up or bends forward it can dig into the upper abdomen or chest, causing pain. It frequently crumbles and plaster falls down inside the cast and also onto the bed. This causes itching and discomfort.

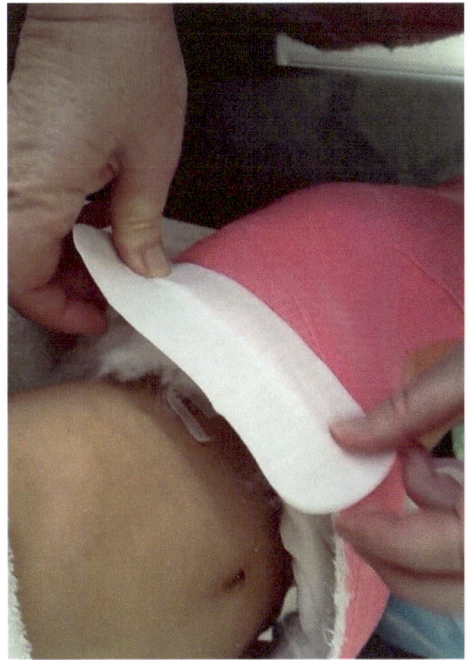 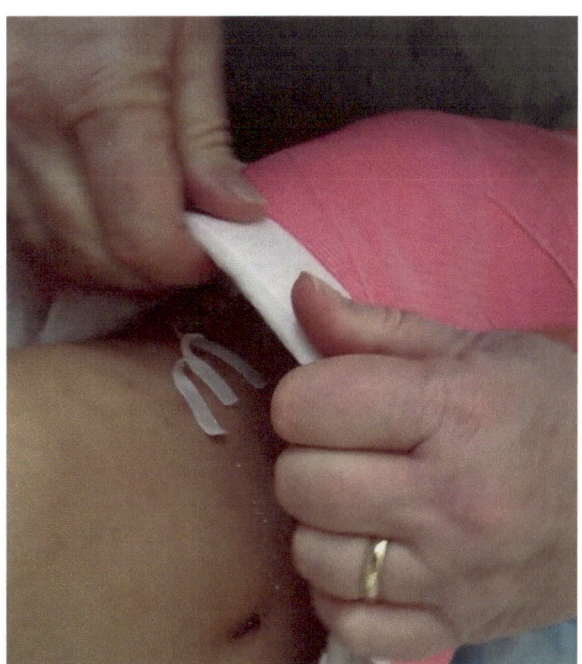

To counteract these issues, panty liners can be used to line the edge of the cast.

TIP! They are an inexpensive alternative to the waterproof tape and also softer and easier to replace. They are also useful in absorbing sweat and controlling odour.

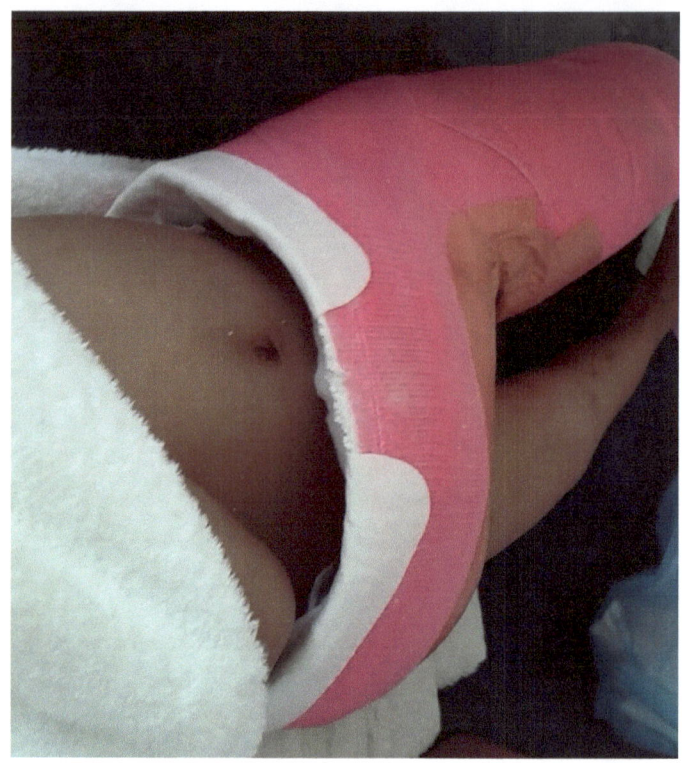

Apply panty liners to the sides of the cast first and fold under, pressing firmly to stick.

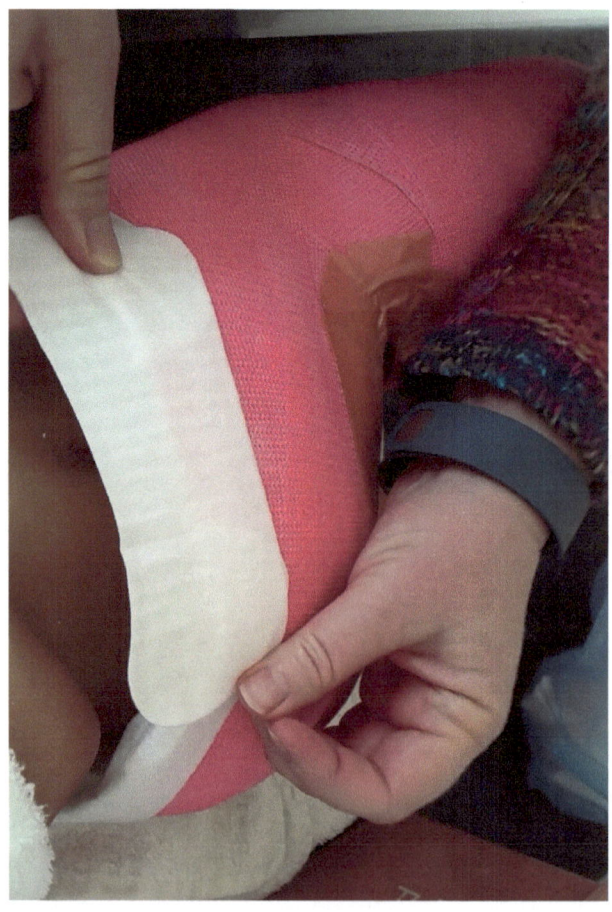

Then stick another panty liner over the middle section and fold under firmly.

TIP! This liner holds the side ones in place and prevents the edges from lifting.

18

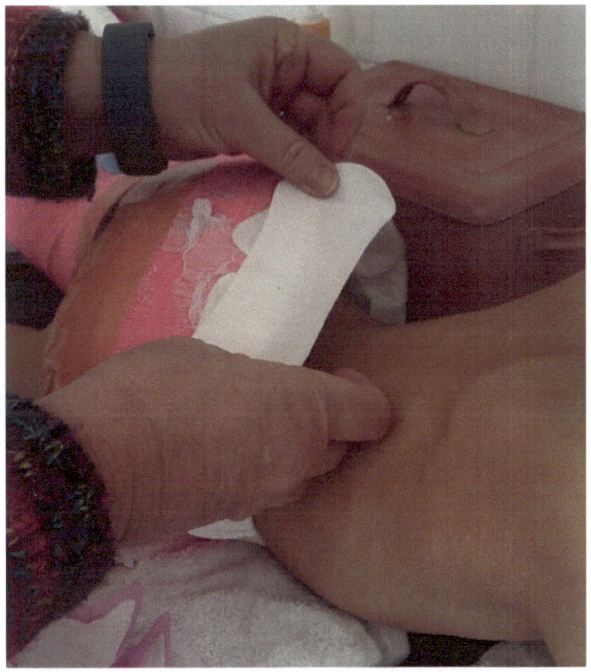

Roll your child onto their stomach and repeat on the back the same as for the front.

TIP! The panty liners on the back usually have to be changed more often, simply because the child is on their back more and they tend to roll up more easily.

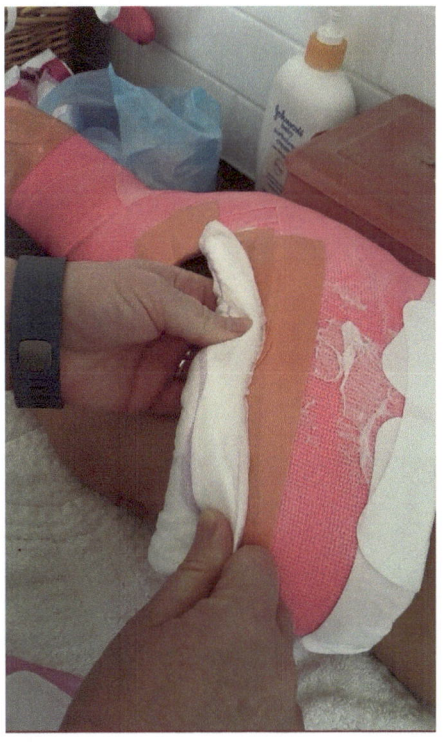

If you feel you would like to use panty liners over the taped buttock and groin areas, as an added protection or simply for comfort, feel free to do so. Indeed in the early days, when there are more accidents, an incontinence pad may be used on the edges.

TIP! When using panty liners on the buttock and groin areas, ensure you still have the medical tape underneath to prevent the plaster becoming wet from urine.

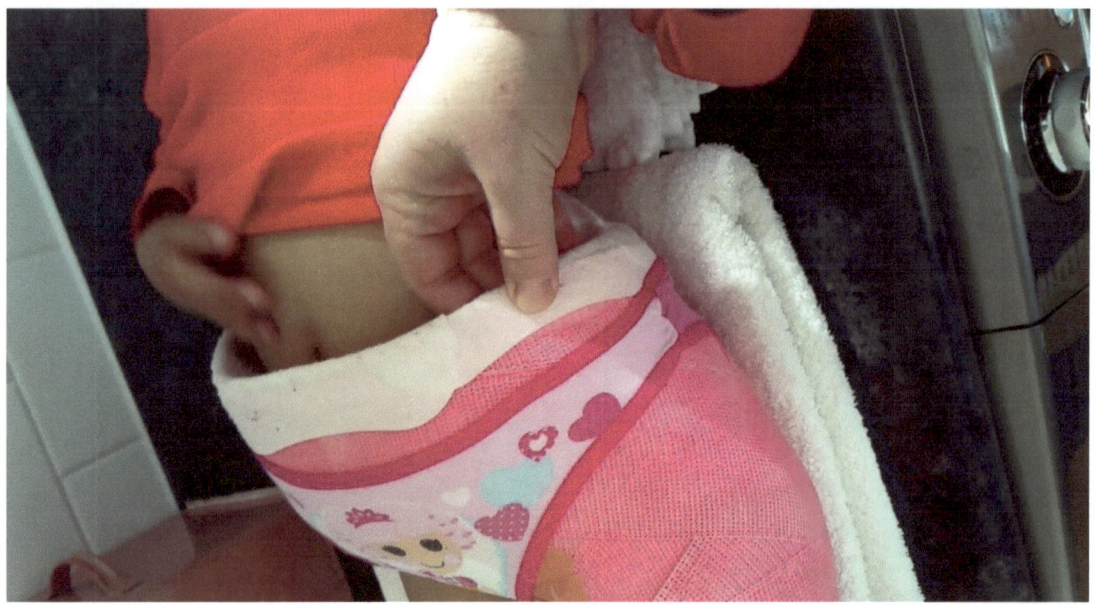

Unless soiled or peeling up, the panty liners can stay in place for a number of days.

TIP! When the panty liners start to pill or ball, take this as an indicator to change them.

TIP! The panty liners help deter plaster crumbs falling but occasionally a few escape. If you see plaster crumbs, particularly just under the cast, flick them out.

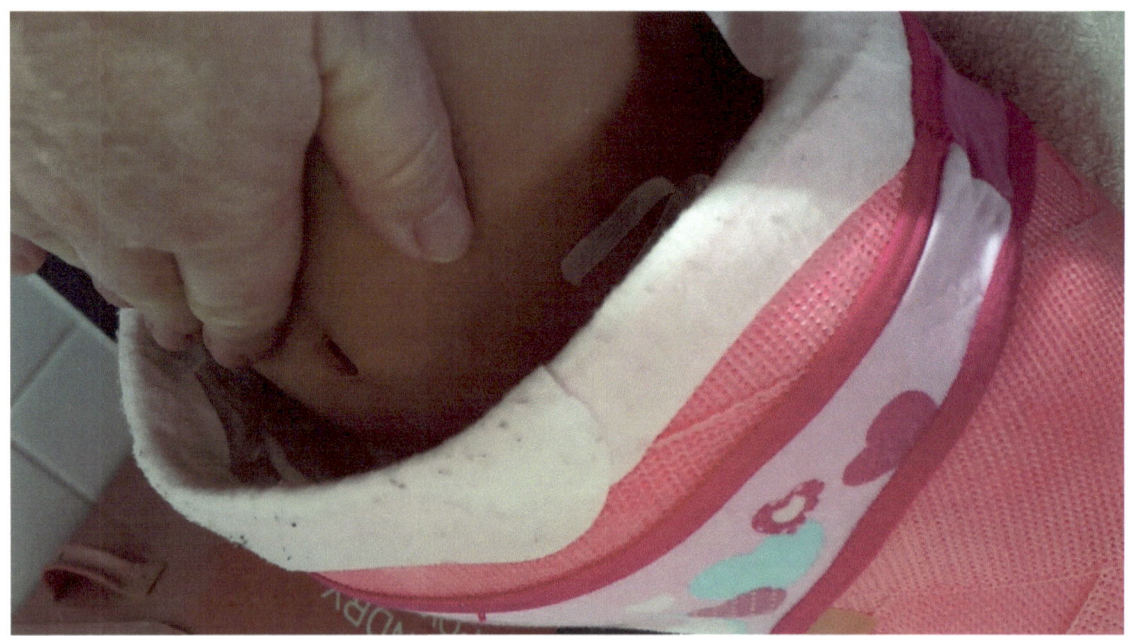

SAFETY TIP! Some children like to hide toys, food, pencils etc., inside their cast. If left inside the cast it can cause pain, discomfort and sometimes infection. Always inspect the inside of your childs cast daily for foreign objects, particularly if your child is complaining that something is hurting them.

If the item is close enough to retrieve safely and is not near the wound, then do so. If the item has gone too far inside the cast to retrieve or is near the wound then take your child to a clinic and let the doctor or practice nurse do it for you. If you cannot see anything and your child is still in pain then the cast may need to be removed, in a hospital, for further investigation. In this case, contact your child's surgeon.

PROTECTING THE INSIDE OF THE CAST

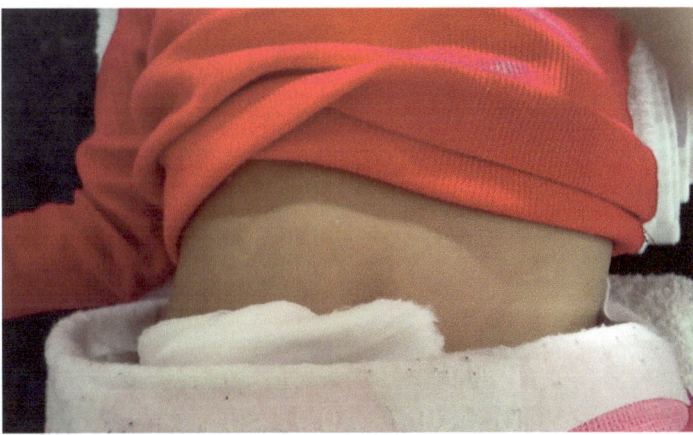 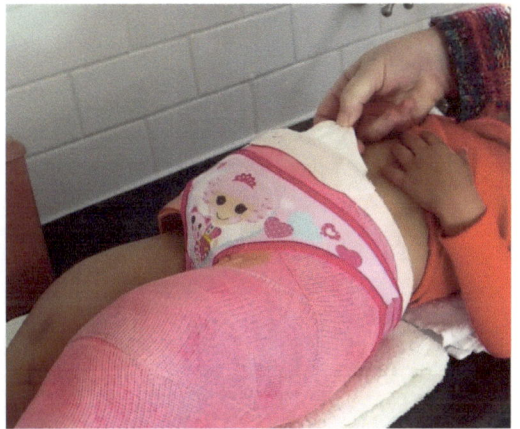

If the cotton wool wadding under the cast becomes wet with urine or soiled with faeces, REMOVE IT. If you leave faeces behind it will create bacteria, smell and cause irritation. If there is residual faeces on the inside of the cast, remove as much as possible with a well wrung out, damp wash cloth.

SAFETY TIP! Only go inside the cast as far as the second joint of your finger and stay away from the wound area. If the wound is covered in faeces then contact your surgeon. He may well want to replace the cast to avoid infection.

TIP! You will need to replace the cotton wool wadding with something to use as a comfort barrier between the cast and the skin. Incontinence or even slightly thicker menstrual pads work very well in these areas as they are soft, absorb sweat and urine and also contain an odour absorbing component. Try to only use unscented pads as scented ones may irritate sensitive skin.

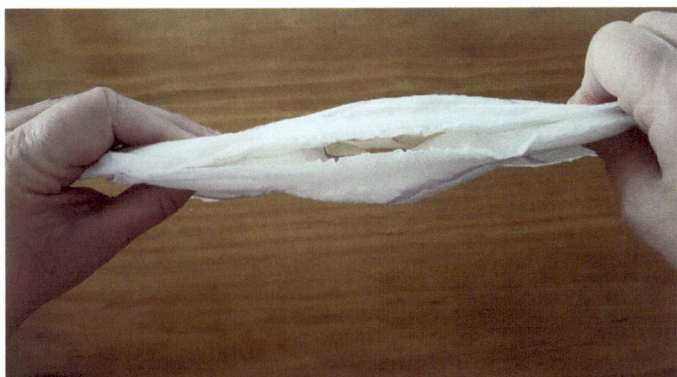 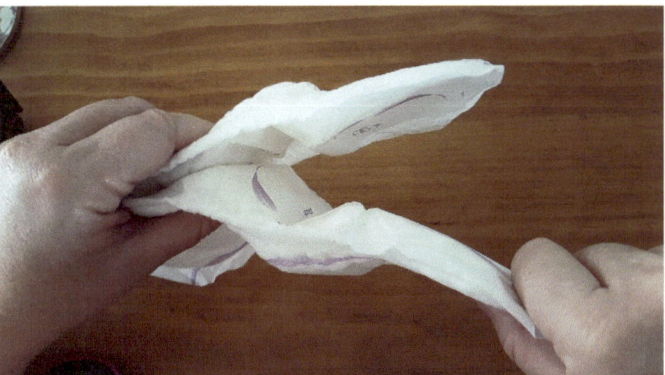

Take two incontinence or menstrual pads and place them back to back.

TIP! Ensure you have the adhesive sides touching each other. You can stick the two pads together if you wish or leave the tabs in place and simply place together. If you choose to stick them together you will have to replace both when one becomes soiled whereas if you don't stick them you only have to replace the soiled one.

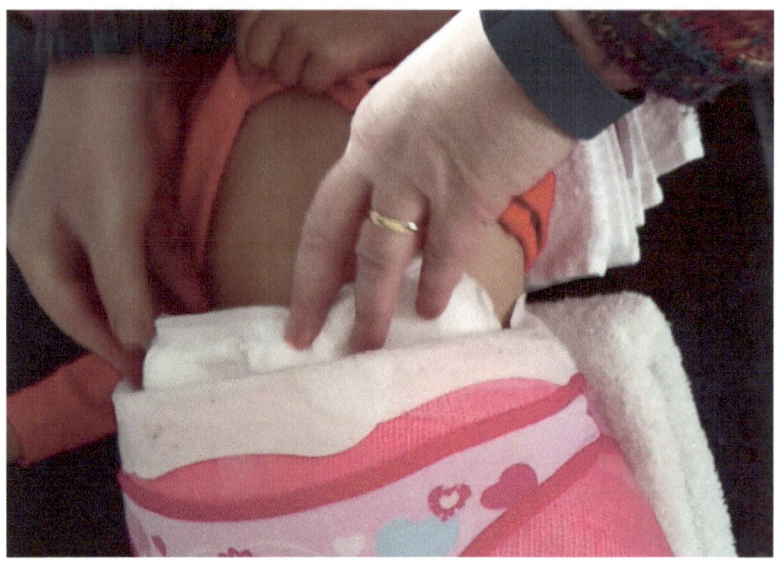

Slide the two back to back pads into place together. Repeat in the back area. After first inserting the pads after soiling, change at least twice a day till all moisture and odour has gone. You will only have to change as required after this point.

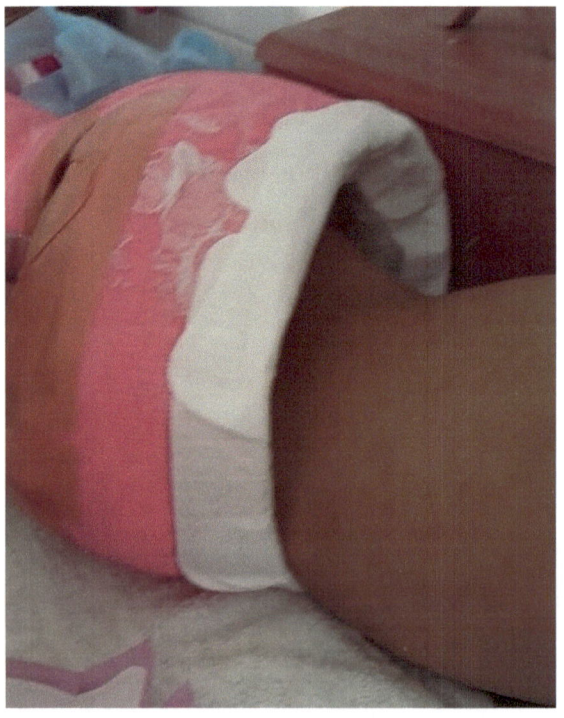

Roll your child onto their tummy and repeat the same as for the front by removing the wadding and replacing with two incontinence pads back to back.

TIP! This padding provides more comfort when on their back as well as absorbing sweat and urine.

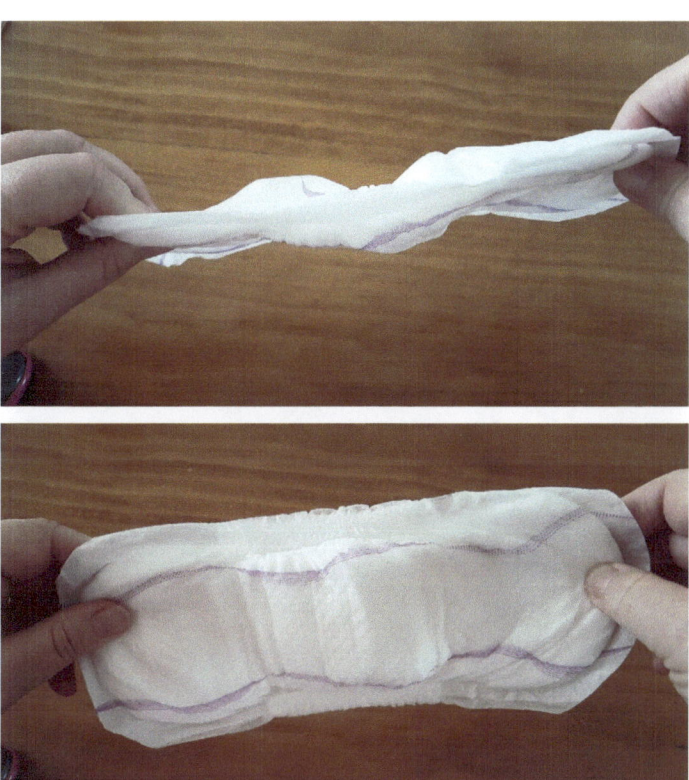

Incontinence pads or larger menstrual pads can be used to cover the groin area. This is to prevent little accidents becoming bigger ones.

TIP! The pad only needs to be changed if it becomes soiled or begins to smell therefore saving money. In the case of a child that uses the toilet it can last all day.

TIP! Always use a fresh pad after a wash.

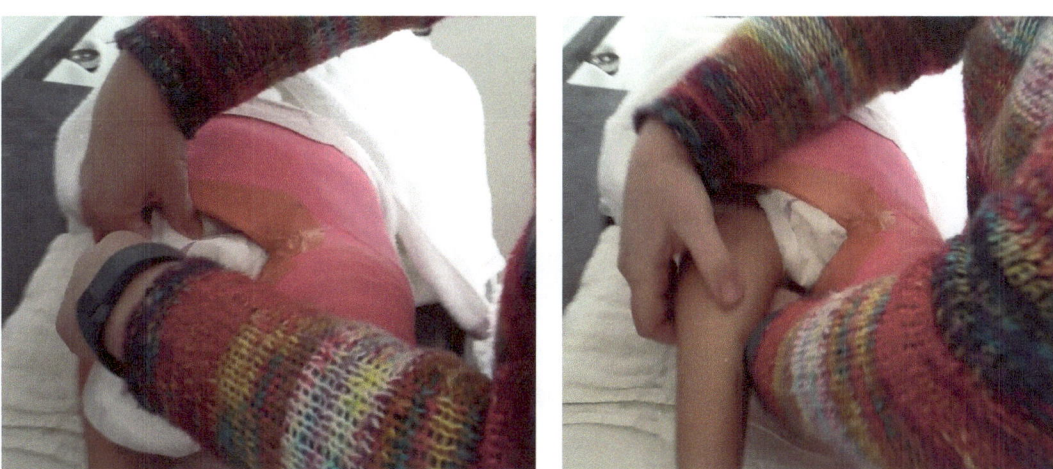

Using only one pad this time, push one end up under the cast, fold it right under the genital and anal area and if the child is small it can also be tucked in under the back of the cast.

TIP! A nappy may also be used in the same manner but the adhesive tabs do not need to be used.

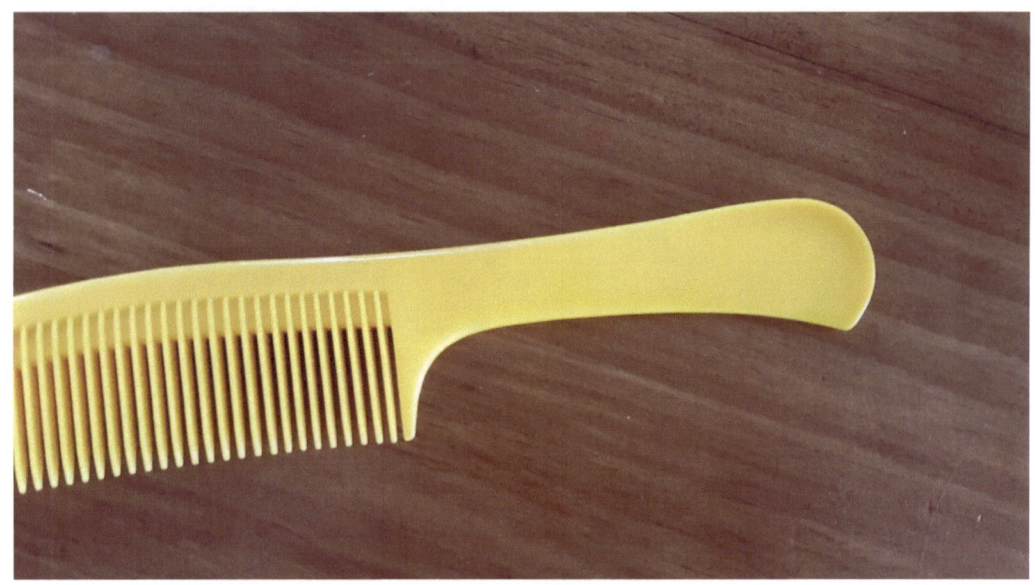

TIP! A flat, broad handled comb serves well to push an incontinence pad or nappy up under the cast when there is minimal room for your fingers; for example, when the cast is tighter. Ensure that there are no sharp edges on the comb handle or any other implement you decide to use.

SAFETY TIP! Remember to stay away from the wound area with the comb or other item you use to push the pads in.

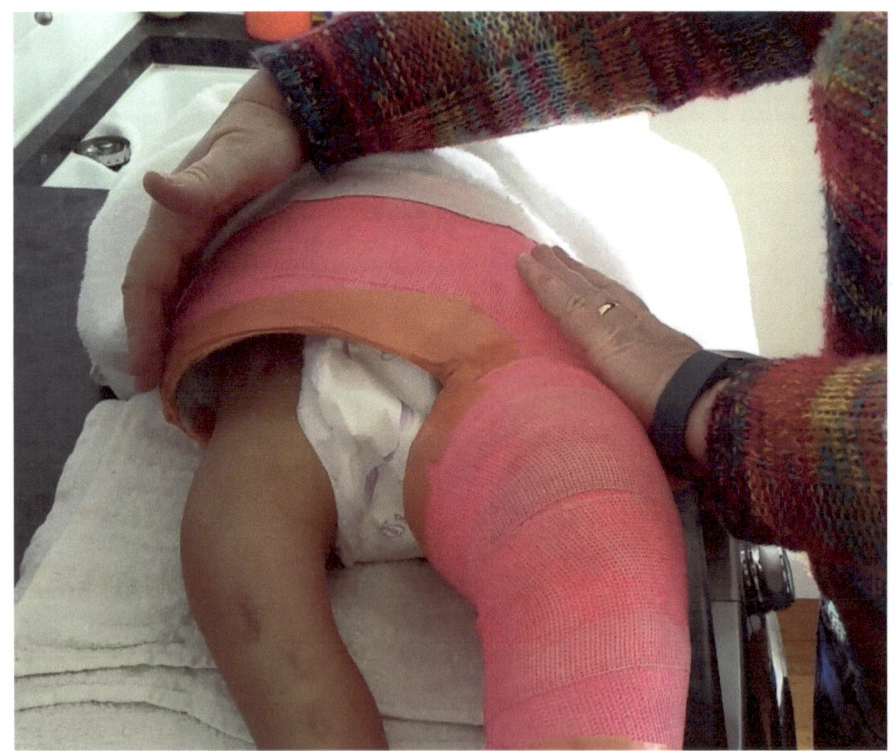

After the pad or nappy has been inserted under the cast you will need something to hold it in place.

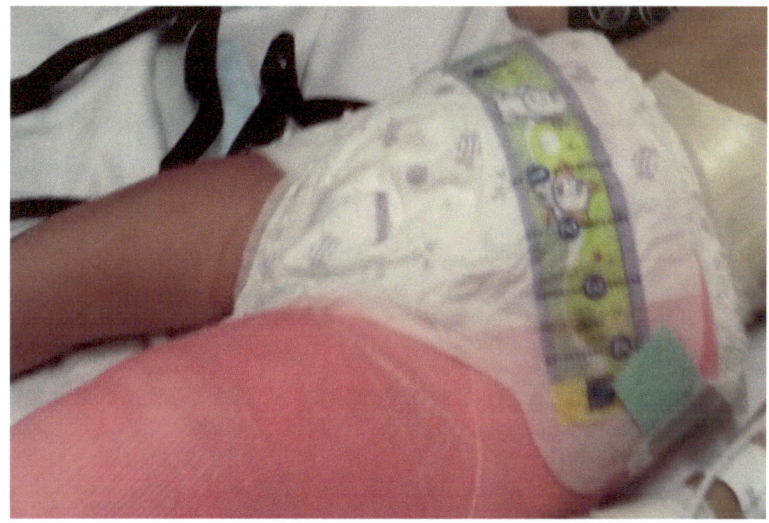

Extra-large nappies work extremely well in this area and can be used on babies, toddlers as well as older children who have taken a little step back in their toilet training due to surgery and the resultant pain.

TIP! Toilet training regression is only a minor setback and will come back in time. No need to stress.

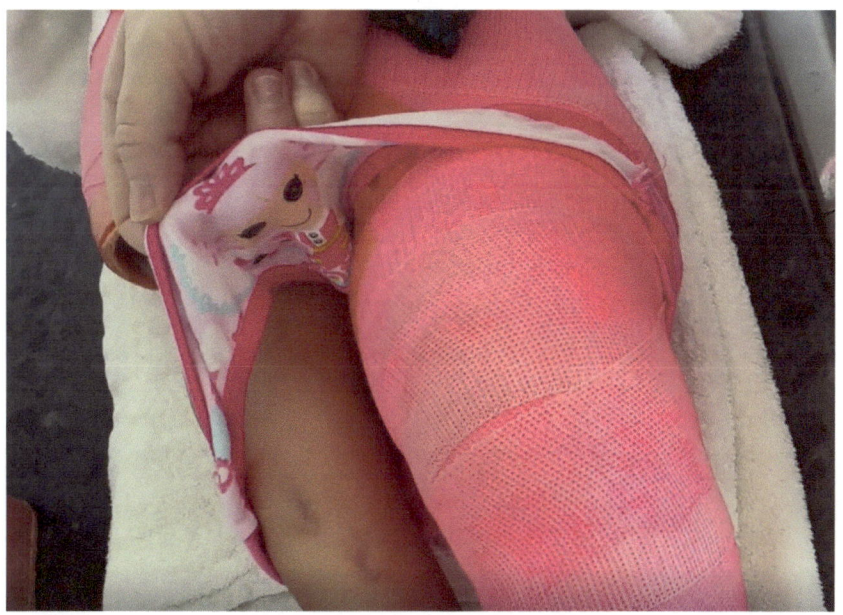

Underpants can be used to cover the pad to hold it in place. Make sure you buy several sizes larger to be able to accommodate the size of the hip spica.

TIP! Don't purchase expensive underwear as the rough fiberglass covering tends to shred them fairly quickly.

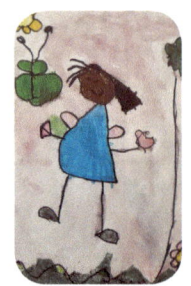

TOILETING

When toileting, it comes down to whether you feel your child can cope going to the toilet either with or without your help (depending on age and ability). Some children regress and go back into nappies whilst others prefer to toilet from day one. Some children wear a nappy just in case of accidents but prefer to use the toilet. Remember to not stress as their toileting skills will return.

Small children can be lifted onto the seat and either held in position or if they practice enough can hold themselves in position. Use of a toilet-potty seat may help some for stability if the cast is small enough and the shape will allow.

SAFETY TIP! Children should never be left on the toilet alone.

SAFETY TIP! Boys will have to sit down to use the toilet unless they are strong enough to stand on one leg to urinate and if that leg is not in a cast. Although for younger and smaller boys the weight of the cast can cause them to overbalance and topple over.

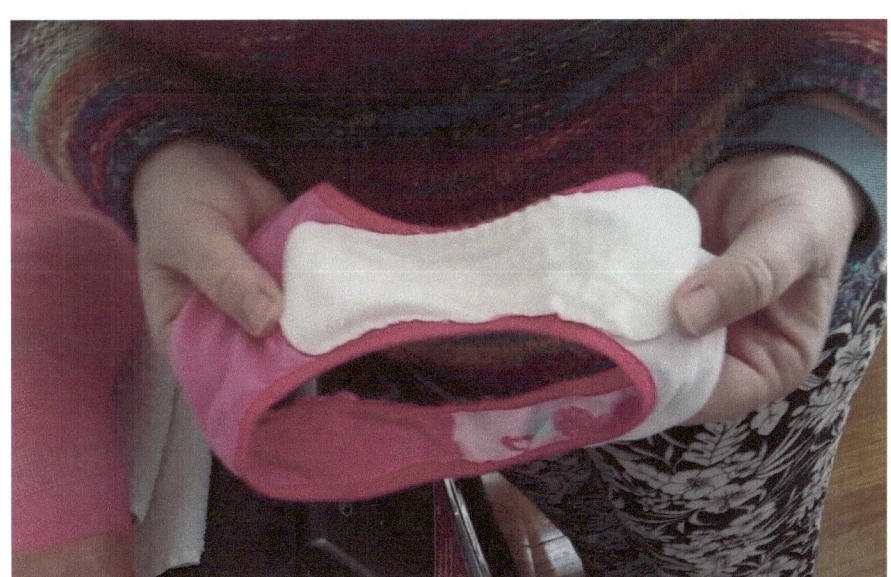

If your child is managing toileting well and can hold their bladder till they make it to the toilet then you may use a panty liner instead of the bulkier incontinence pad. This contains little dribbles if they happen.

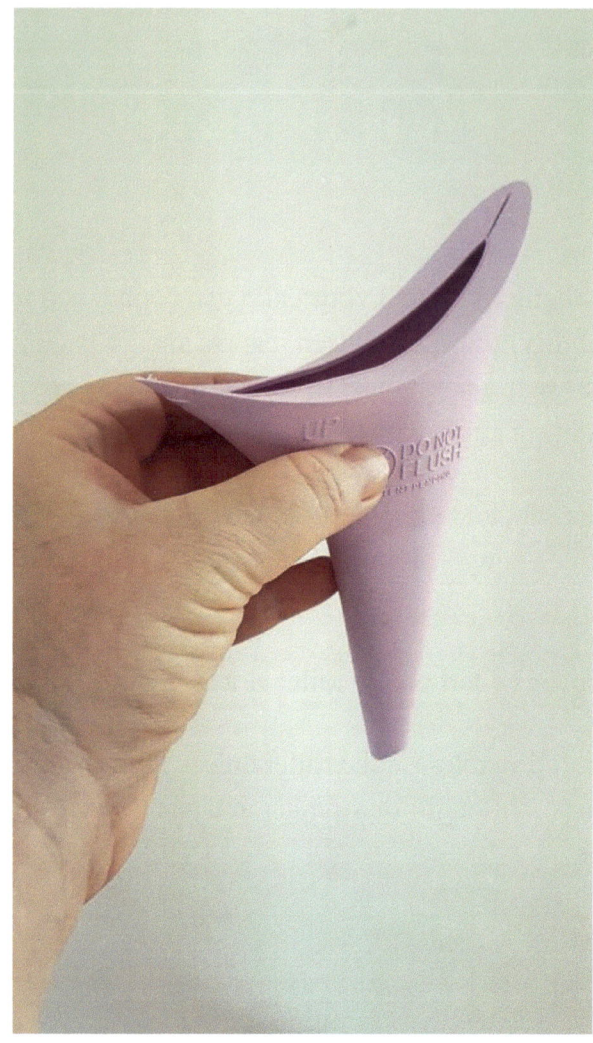

Any child, regardless of gender can use a toilet can use an aid (pictured). It is helpful in making sure the stream goes into the toilet and not on the cast. Small accidents may occur when practicing at first, so prepare with extra padding protection before proceeding.

Once the use of it has been mastered it will save a lot of money and effort as you won't need to use as many incontinence pads or nappies. The aid must be turned around in the opposite direction from the normal way it is supposed to be used but each person has their own individual way of doing it. Stick with what you are comfortable with. These aids trade under various names but are relatively inexpensive to buy online and are reusable, washable silicon in several colours.

TIP! Make sure you practice a lot at home before attempting to use when out.

TIP! They are great to take out with you as they can be washed and popped back into a zip lock bag ready for the next time.

TIP! When purchasing online, search for female urination devices. For more information on the pictured aid there is a website address link in the acknowledgement at the front of this book.

MAKING YOUR CHILD COMFORTABLE

There are a many ways to make your child comfortable whilst in a hip spica. It will depend mainly on what your child prefers so play around with a few things to see what works best.

SAFETY TIP! Encourage your child to move a little from side to side on the pillow or bean bag to promote circulation in their bottom area and relieve pressure. On the bed or floor, encourage your child to roll over onto their tummy as this is also useful to relieve pressure.

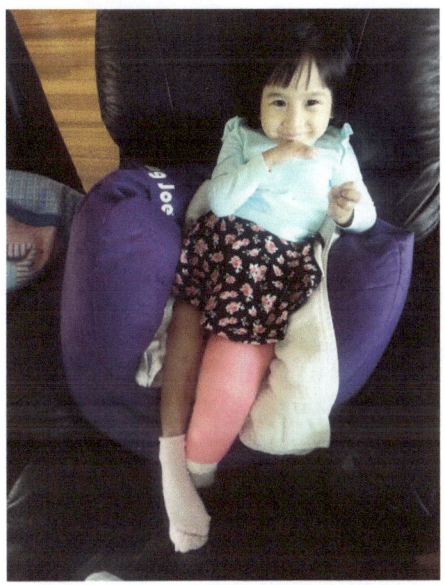

TIP! A bean bag is very useful and can be molded to fit even the most unusually shaped hip spica cast. Small child size versions are available. They are particularly useful when your child wants to sit up to eat as can fit in a dining chair. A chair with arms works better.

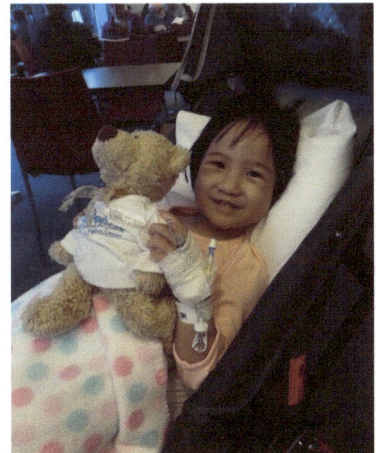

TIP! A large stroller/jogger can double as a chair when you child wishes to sit up. For example it can be used when watching television or at a table to eat.

TIP! Pillows and cushions are very useful for getting your child into a comfortable position. In the picture above, one pillow was placed under the child's bottom and legs and another down behind the head, neck and back (both pillows lengthways).

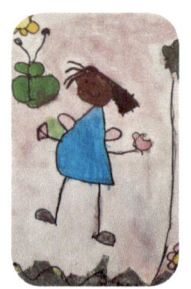

CLOTHING

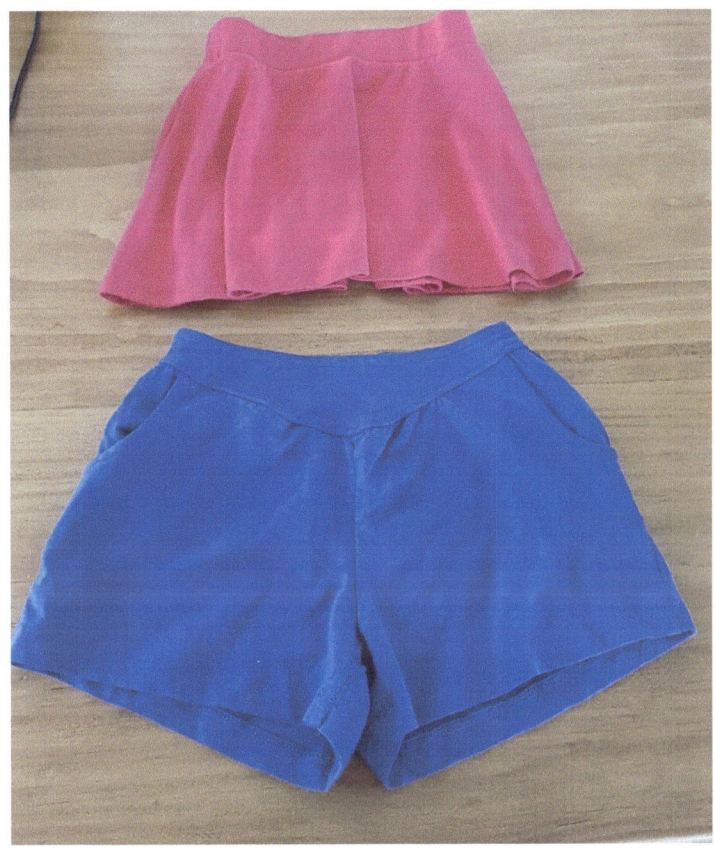

When dressing your child it is better to have clothing that is loose fitting for easy removal. It also makes going to the toilet or nappy changing much easier. For girls, skirts are great and for both boys and girls, shorts or track pants work well. You will have to get clothing that is larger round the middle to accommodate the wide girth of the hip spica. Underwear needs to be several sizes larger to accommodate the cast too.

TIP! As a rule of thumb, buy clothing that is several sizes larger than they would ordinarily wear.

TIP! Children are usually only in a hip spica anywhere between six weeks to twelve weeks. To reduce costs some people prefer not to buy expensive clothing for their children during that time. Once out of the cast the clothes will not fit.

TIP! The legs on shorts and track pants need to be extra wide.

TIP! Make sure your child's feet are kept warm enough, particularly in a cooler climate. As your child is unable to move the casted leg or foot very much their circulation is not that of a normally mobile child and is therefore reduced. Encourage your child to wiggle their feet and toes as much as possible. Cover their feet with socks or a small blanket.

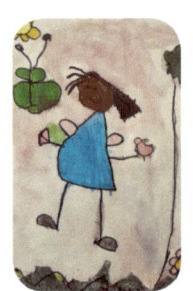

MOBILITY

Smaller children are quite adept at dragging themselves around a floor to get to a toy or activity. Their determination won't be waned by the weight of the hip spica; it is merely a challenge. A soft blanket underneath can help.

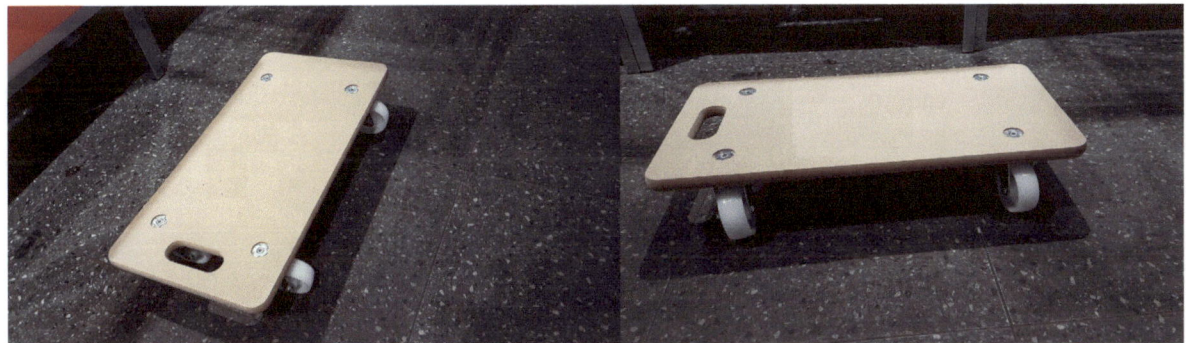

However, if you don't want the hip spica damaged or dirty from the floor then a dolley will work wonders. They have the added advantage of being close to the floor, so if your child does roll off they shouldn't hurt themselves. It will also save your floors being scratched or carpet shredded by the cast. Make sure the wheels are large enough to go over all surfaces e.g. carpet, wood flooring and tiles. They are an inexpensive helper that allows your child to move about themselves. Dolley's can be purchased for as low as $20. They are available from hardware stores and some supermarkets.

TIP! Some dolley's, depending on wheel size, can be used outside on concrete or grass which gives your child some much needed outdoor time.

TIP! If you are a bit of a handyman/handywoman then have a go making one. Ensure that is strong enough to take the weight of the child and hip spica and that there are no sharp edges on the platform. Ensure the wheels are large enough to roll over carpet.

SAFETY TIP! Please make sure you watch where your child is at all times. As they are low to the ground, they are not easy to see. Be careful not to stand on or trip over them.

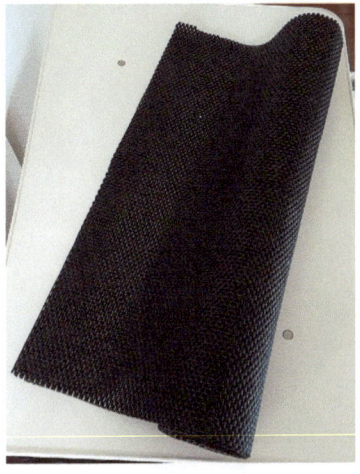

SAFETY TIP! Put a non-slip mat on the top of the dolley so the child does not slip off when scooting about.

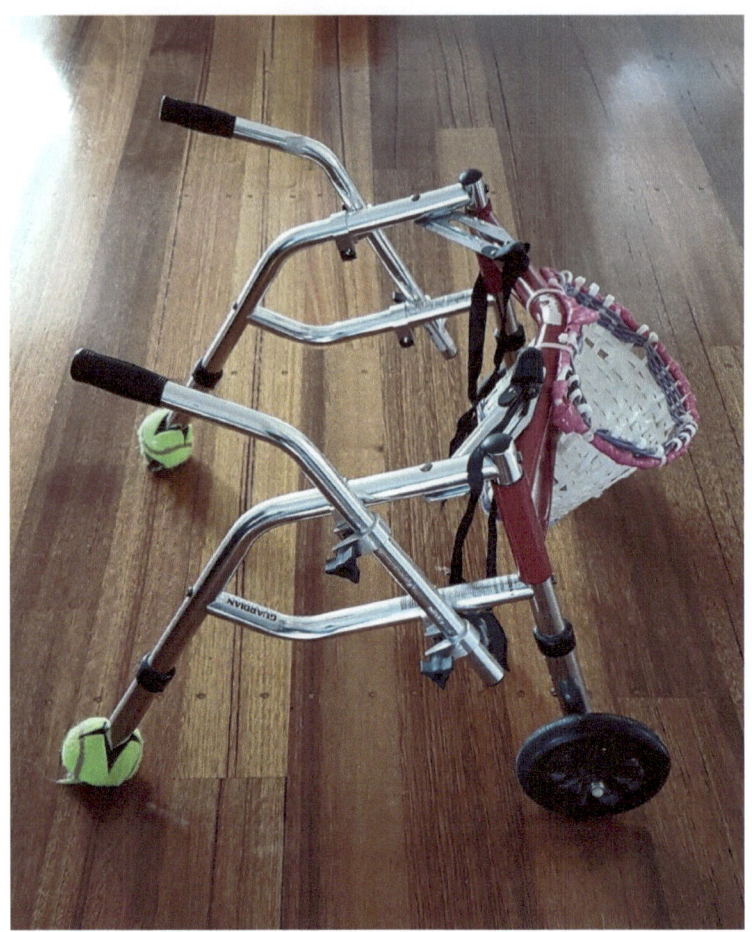

An alternative for moving around is a walker. Some hospitals will loan them to your child and give lessons from a therapist on how to walk with one. If this service is not offered then you can find your own therapist who, usually, will arrange walker hire for you.

SAFETY TIP! The foot in the cast is usually non-weight bearing so should not rest on the ground when moving about.

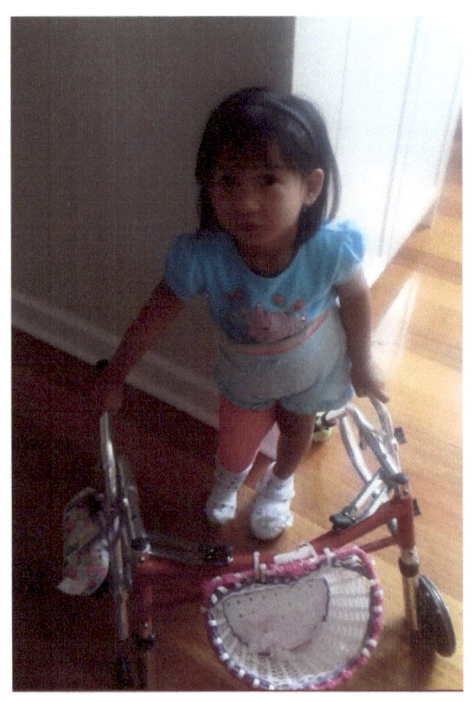

CAR SEATS

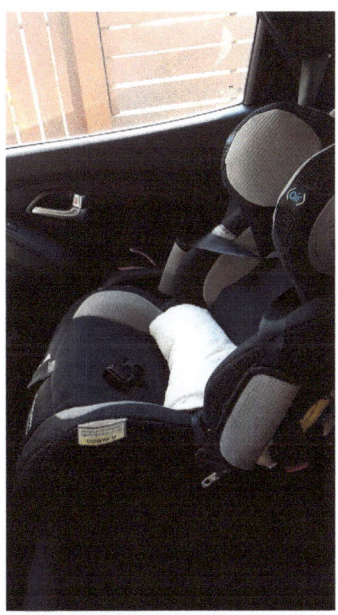

Car seats can be made comfortable with the use of towels or a wedge of foam rubber placed behind your child's lower back.

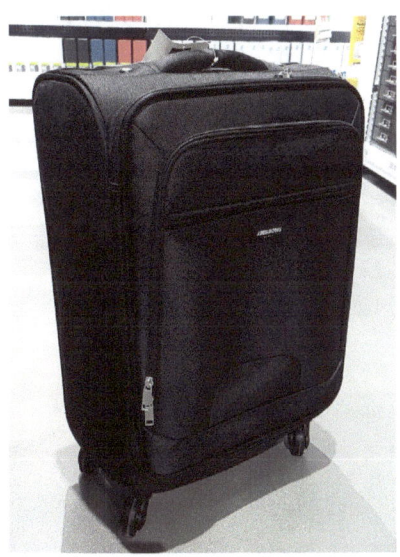

Support of the leg (that is casted) in the car is essential as the weight of the cast can pull the leg down. This will make your child uncomfortable and they will constantly work hard to try and keep the leg up.

TIP! This can be avoided by using a strong carry-on wheelie case or other strong box-like item under their foot and ankle. As long as it is at a height that keeps the leg level with their hip. Place a towel or soft padding on top of the case, to rest on and to prevent the leg from sliding off.

TIP! Older and taller children can sit in the centre seat and place their foot on the central console between the two front seats. Again their foot and ankle should be resting on soft padding for comfort.

SAFETY TIP! All children should be in approved seat belts whilst in a car.

TIP! Encourage your child to wiggle their bottom occasionally to increase circulation.

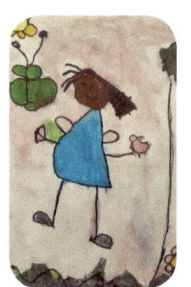

CONCLUSION

There are a great many ways of completing tasks and caring for your child in a hip spica cast that can work. This guide suggests ways of undertaking necessary tasks that may help parents cope better with caring for their child whilst in a hip spica cast.

These suggestions are not fixed in stone so may be adapted or changed to suit the parent's or carers needs. Always remember, safety first to reduce the risk of injury to both yourself and your child.

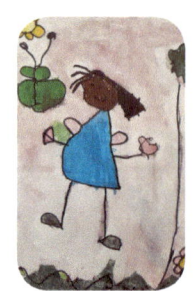

ABOUT THE AUTHOR

Robyn Lambert is from Geelong in the state of Victoria, Australia where she lives with the love of her life. Robyn has four amazing children who have all, with their distinctive personalities, inspired her writing.

Robyn has worked as a nurse for over 20 years and also studied Anthropology, Language and Culture. She also has a personal interest in children's special needs. Robyn likes to incorporate not only cultural differences in her books but differences that make us all unique and interesting individuals.

www.ingramcontent.com/pod-product-compliance
Lightning Source LLC
Chambersburg PA
CBHW041523280526
45792CB00004B/1358